When opposites attract...
Sex matters

When opposites attract...
Sex matters

Steve Chalke and
Nick Page

Hodder & Stoughton
LONDON SYDNEY AUCKLAND

First published in Great Britain 1996.

10 9 8 7 6 5 4 3 2 1

British Library Cataloguing in Publication Data
A record for this book is available from the British Library.

ISBN 0 340 65661 1

Designed and typeset by Typograph, Irby, Wirral, Cheshire.
Printed and bound in Great Britain by Cox & Wyman Ltd, Reading, Berkshire

Hodder and Stoughton Ltd,
A division of Hodder Headline PLC
338 Euston Road, London NW1 3BH

Contents

Thanks to
Paul and *James*,
and the many, many other people
who helped us write this book.
Thanks especially to *Claire* and *Cornelia*,
who gave us lots of practical help as well!

1

It's a sex-mad world

'SIX STEPS to hot summer sex.'

'Ultimate sex test: how will your lover score?'

'Falling in love . . . how to know when you are ready to go all the way!'

'Knickers to get you noticed.'

'Orgasms: a girl's guide to toe-curling, spine-tingling, back-arching bliss!'

Forget the top shelf. These are all genuine front cover captions from best-selling magazines, written for the teenage market and available in any high street store.

Sex is everywhere

The old Victorian era, in which sex was the Great Unmentionable, is dead and gone. And you don't have to look too far for the evidence. Sex is everywhere.

A few years ago, if you were one of the lucky ones, your father or mother would sit you down for 'that talk'. Each side dreaded it. In fact, parents usually found it far more embarrassing than their children. Most parents, however, were too embarrassed even to mention it.

Nowadays, it's more likely that a son or daughter has to sit their parent or parents down and ask them straight: 'Mum, dad . . . is there anything you want to know about sex? Don't feel shy. Now's the time to ask!'

And how do young people get to know so much more about sex than their parents did at their age? Simple: it's everywhere.

We'll be right back, after this word . . .

It's in the adverts.

It's used to sell cars, perfume, drink, food, clothes and magazines. In fact, it's used to sell almost anything. Which means, of course, that the products often have nothing whatsoever to do with sex.

The ironic thing is that when condoms were first advertised on television in 1987, the ads contained high-wire fences and lots of very anxious teenagers, but less sexual excitement than the average chocolate bar commercial.

In two of the most amazing ad campaigns of the last few years, everyone was talking about the Gold Blend couples. The ads were nothing to do with coffee. All the public were interested in was: Were the couple going to get together? Were they going to kiss? Would they end up in bed?

Ice-cream adverts feature women sensuously losing their clothing, and perfectly formed semi-naked people eating Maple Nut Crunch in positions that would make a contortionist weep.

Ordinary men become sexual magnets to beautiful women when they splash on that irresistible 'Woman Killer' aftershave, or get behind the wheel of a new Brand X car.

It just proves that sex can be used to sell anything.

'This week: 19,642 ways to satisfy your partner'

It's in the newspapers and magazines.

The tabloids use sex to boost sales and attract readers. Since he took it over and introduced the Page Three topless model, media mogul Rupert Murdoch has made *The Sun* the biggest-selling daily newspaper in the UK by a long way. And the top shelf in most newsagents is crammed with pornographic magazines.

Well-known magazines like *Mizz*, *Just 17* and *More*, as well as *Cosmopolitan* and *Vogue*, are increasingly explicit in their coverage of sex. No month's copy is complete, it seems, without an article or two on 'How to get and keep your man' or 'Fifteen different sexual postions for a Monday morning'. Two lines telling you that you don't have to have sex if you don't want to are overwhelmed by two pages of positions, penises and penetration .

'Get on the scene . . . lile a sex machine . . .'

Sex is in the charts.

Sex has always been part of rock and pop music. In the 1950s, Elvis Presley's 'gyrating' hips were banned from American TV screens because outraged parents believed they would prove too sexually stimulating for their innocent daughters.

The Beatles showed beyond doubt that rock and pop have never just been about songs. When they gave concerts in the 1960s, at the peak of 'Beatlemania', young women would scream so loudly at the thrill of being in the same building as the Fab Four that it was virtually impossible to hear the music.

Nowadays, however, we've entered a different league. Elvis's hips seem positively tame. And it's hard to think of anyone being reduced to jelly today over The Beatles' suits and hairstyles.

Sexually explicit lyrics are part and parcel of every other pop song, whilst stars frequently pose in varying states of undress. If 1950s parents objected to Elvis's swinging hips, what would they make of the world of pelvic thrusts and groin-clutching?

'He took her in his strong and powerful arms, and she knew this was heaven . . .'

Sex is in the bestseller lists.

Sex has always sold books. Many of Shakespeare's plays were raunchy and crammed full with sexual comments. *The Merry Wives of Windsor*, for instance, is the mother of all *Carry On* films. And things got far steamier after Shakespeare's death, when women were allowed to act on stage.

D. H. Lawrence's novel, *Lady Chatterley's Lover*, was banned in the UK for 35 years for its blatant sexual content.

Today Jackie Collins, Jilly Cooper, Sidney Sheldon and other such writers rely heavily on sex to spice up their books. Even Mills & Boon, famous for their romantic page-turners, have become saucier over the last few years. And Virgin (rather inappropriately!) has published Black Lace, a range of erotic fiction aimed at female readers.

Bump and Grind: The Movie (Cert. 18)

And of course, sex is on the TV and in the movies.

Hollywood used to have a rule that either the man or the woman or both had to have at least one foot on the floor during any love scene. For the major studios, any nudity was definitely out.

When it was released in 1934, *It Happened One Night* produced a scandal. Self-appointed watchdogs of public morality were in absolute outrage. Why? Because of one scene in which, pretending to be married, leading man Clark Gable and leading woman Claudette Colbert share a bedroom (though not a bed), dressed only in their pyjamas and separated by a blanket hung over a washing line!

Nowadays, few self-respecting films or TV dramas seem to come without at least one fully-fledged, totally naked, sweat-inducing, eyeball-popping, spectacle-misting sex scene, complete with the moans, groans and heavy breathing of a Nicam Digital Stereo full vocal accompaniment.

Although, in theory, there is supposed to be a nine o'clock 'watershed', sex is everywhere almost all the time. In the early-evening soaps, teenagers discuss, not whether they should be 'doing it', but when, with whom and how many times a week.

And it is virtually impossible to walk around Blockbuster or your local video store without coming face to face with half a dozen steamy tales of sex, secrecy, stockings and suspenders. Even if what you were really looking for was Bugs Bunny!

One way or the other, it seems, we're surrounded by sex.

Questions

- Why do you think sex is such a big seller in society today?
- Do you think that you are affected by the amount of sex on show?
- Do you think there should be more, or less, sex in books and magazines and on TV? Why?

12

2

Decisions, decisions . . .

WITH ALL THIS information bombarding us, it is easy to think that there is no life before sex.

'You've read the book, you've seen the film, you've heard the soundtrack, you've got the T-shirt, now go out and do it!' This is the message that is pumped at us non-stop.

Sex must be the most important thing in the world. Otherwise why would it be promoted so much? It's obvious that until we have had sex we are nothing and nobody. We feel that until we've 'done it', we're not really mature – we haven't *arrived*.

Sex is rather like shaving, or wearing your first bra. It's seen as a kind of 'badge' of adulthood. Somehow we feel that if we haven't yet started slapping on the shaving foam or strapping on an 'over-the-shoulder boulder-holder', then we aren't as much of a man or woman as those of our friends who have. It can make us feel very left out. And it's the same with sex.

Sex is often seen as the natural next step after puberty.

And if everyone else is 'doing it', we don't want to be left behind. We don't want to be the only one who can't boast about who we 'got off' with on holiday or at a party on Saturday night.

But is that a good reason for having sex?

Do the right thing

A lot of people start smoking because everyone else is doing it. It's the cool thing to do. The adult thing to do. Maybe even the 'sexy' thing to do. But all this doesn't even begin to make it the *right* thing to do.

The truth is, of course, that the decision to start smoking has big consequences. It can give you lung cancer, heart disease, cancer of the mouth, bronchitis, emphysema and even gangrene. Not to mention yellow-stained hands and teeth. How sexy is that? And, most important of all, it can make you even less pleasant to kiss than a camel with bad breath.

Everyone else may be doing it, but is that really a good reason to start smoking? And it's just the same when it comes to sex. Even if everyone else were doing it, it would still make a lot of sense for you carefully to consider the implications and consequences of taking such an important step. Are you absolutely sure that it's the right thing for you to do now? Is it a step you're certain you are ready to take?

Appearances are deceptive

Wouldn't it be terrible to have sex before you really wanted to – before you felt ready and before you felt that it was 'right' – just because you didn't want to be the odd one out, only to discover that people you *thought* had had sex, actually *hadn't*?

Yet that's exactly what happens to some people.

Mizz magazine appeals to the more sexually aware teenager. But a survey of its readers revealed that whilst 49 per cent had had sex before the age of 16, as many as 85 per cent thought that their friends and peers had had sex before this age.

'*It's official*,' they concluded, '*other people have sex later than you think!*'

Just like the first time

So choose your moment carefully, because first impressions count. Many people's attitude to sex is conditioned, or at least coloured, by their first time.

For some people, this will have been planned and prepared for – maybe even long-hoped for – with the moment, the partner, the location and the atmosphere chosen with care.

For a great many, however, the first time will not provide such a pleasant memory. It will have happened when they didn't really want it or feel ready, but felt it was something they had to do, because either their friends or their partner was pushing them to do it.

According to the Family Planning Association (FPA), one in every fifteen women between the ages of 15 and 19 gets pregnant. But the shock is that the FPA also estimates that some 90 per cent of these get pregnant unintentionally. And even more surprisingly, most of them did not intend even to have sex in the first place, much less a baby!

A small number of these women will have been raped or abused, but the great majority will either have been pressured by their boyfriend into agreeing to have sex when they didn't want to, or else simply have been overtaken by the passion of the moment, only later to regret their actions.

And it's not just girls who end up having sex when they don't really want to. Many a guy has got carried away in the heat of passion, only to regret his actions later. And of course, if you're at a party and you've had a few drinks, it's amazing how attractive you can find someone you normally think of as being about as sexy as the Elephant Man! You're in serious danger of waking up the next morning wondering why on earth you did *that* with *them!*

'I'll know what I think just as soon as someone tells me'

The truth is that sex is important.

That means it's not something we should treat lightly or casually: it should be treated with respect. To make love just because the media, the adverts, your friends, or your boyfriend or girlfriend are telling you to do so, is to take something very special and treat it very cheaply.

We all know sex means more than that.

We all want the first time to be special. Memorable. We want to be able to look back, maybe feel some of the same dizzy, tingling sensations again, and think, 'I'm really glad I did that!'

But we are surrounded by sexual messages and images. And although many of them are fake, either selling us something or promising what they can never deliver, they can seem very convincing. So we need to be careful we don't end up simply absorbing them all just like a sponge soaks up water, and letting them distort our understanding of what sex really is.

Don't be pushed into anything. When you *do* have sex – for the first time or any time – it should be for the right reasons, at the right time, and because both you and your partner want to.

Don't compromise. Choose for yourself. Make your own decisions. It's your *right* to do so.

Sex matters. That's why it's special, and worth treating with care.

Questions

- Why do you think people feel the need to lie about having sex?
- In what circumstances have you done things you didn't want to do simply because everyone else was doing them?
- What do you think makes sex with someone you care about different from sex with someone you don't really know?

3

It's only natural

THE FIRST THING TO SAY about sex is that sexuality – everything that makes us male or female – is a *good* thing.

Throughout the centuries, some people have been keen to condemn the whole area of our sexuality. They have pictured it as a secret, shameful part of our characters. A great many famous statues, for instance, feature men and women who are virtually naked. But a large proportion of them have their sexual 'bits' covered with a carefully positioned fig leaf or two. What's really extraordinary is that very few of these statues originally came with fig leaves; in fact, the sculptors would have been horrified by their presence. So how did they get there? They were added later by people who considered that nakedness was 'indecent', and that it was their duty to make things 'more presentable'.

In the eighteenth and nineteenth centuries, it was common for a husband and wife in polite society to have separate bedrooms. Although people were as interested in sex as ever, few would actually admit to *liking* it. 'Of course, it's necessary in order to continue the human race, but it's messy, and best done at night with the lights off!'

Around 1900, a certain Lady Alice Hillingdon summed it all up when she remarked, 'I am happy now that Charles calls on my bedchamber less frequently than of old. As it is, I now endure but two calls a week and when I hear his steps outside my door I lie down on my bed, close my eyes, open my legs and think of England.'

If the 'earth moved' for Lady Hillingdon, she certainly wasn't letting on about it!

By the 1920s and 1930s, the fashion had changed toward 'twin beds': identical single beds placed alongside one another, often with a small bedside table between them. An improvement, but still hardly the height of unfettered passion!

As someone once commented to a teenage boy, 'Sex is dirty, disgusting and degrading. Save it for your wife!'

The REAL reason for getting your eyes tested

But the fact is that our sexuality is a perfectly natural part of who we are. It's not something to be ashamed of, or to try unnaturally to suppress. It's an important part of being human, something which makes us fully alive. Sexuality is everything that makes men men and women women.

Mostly, though, sexuality finds its expression in the things which make men and women different: in the way they think and feel, and particularly in the way they look.

So when you see a member of the opposite sex and think to yourself, *'Corrrrr!'* – that's not 'wrong': it's just good eyesight. Sexual attraction is part of being human, and the most complete expression of this attraction is sexual intercourse.

Hold your horses!

So if sex is good, should we just go out there and get on with it?

Well, just because something is natural or part of us, that doesn't mean that it's always right or healthy to do it. After all, we all have muscles, but that doesn't make it right to go around using them to hit people whenever we feel like it.

Just because the scientists in the film *Jurassic Park* had the technology to clone dinosaurs, it didn't make it a good idea. They were so busy finding out what they could do that they didn't stop to think whether or not they *should* do these things. Of course, in *Jurassic Park*, people's mistakes actually ate them. Fortunately, sexual mistakes are not always so lethal. (Although, as we shall see in the next chapter, because of sexually transmitted diseases and conditions such as AIDS, they *can* be that lethal.)

Still, just because sex is good doesn't mean that every time people *have* sex it's good. Sometimes the consequences of having sex, even between consenting adults, can be very damaging to one or even both of them.

You may feel ready for sex. You may definitely want to have sex. You may feel that you have found the right partner and the right time. You may be sure that no one has pressured you into this decision.

But however 'right' it feels, you have to consider the facts – i.e., what the consequences might be.

Cream cakes and heart disease

Having the ability or desire to do something doesn't mean that it's automatically *right* to go ahead and do it. For our own good, we all have to learn to control our natural desires. In other words, we have to draw a careful line between 'use' and '*ab*use'.

For instance, eating is a good and essential activity. But stuffing yourself silly with chips or chocolate or cream cakes, day after day after day, is not very healthy in the short term, and in the long term can be deadly. Medical research has shown a direct link between bad eating habits and heart disease. Eating the wrong kind of food, or even too much of the right kind of food, can be very damaging to your health. So eating packet after packet after packet of your favourite crisps may make you *feel* good, but the fact is that it won't be *doing* you good.

And it's the same with our sex drive. You have to consider the possible consequences of your actions carefully. Sex is good. Sex is great! But its abuse is destructive. Just like overeating, it can even kill you!

Questions

- Do you think that people today see sex as good or bad?
- Aside from sex and eating, what else can you think of where abuse is destructive?
- Why do you think people ignore the dangers of casual sex?

4

A twist in the tale

WE DON'T HAVE TO look around very hard to find ways in which sex can sometimes have some extremely damaging consequences. There are some very big risks.

Acquired Immune Deficiency Syndrome, or AIDS, got its name in 1983, when it became clear to scientists that it was a recognisable medical condition. When a person has AIDS, it means that their immune system – the body's way of fighting disease – is not functioning properly. AIDS is a condition, not a disease. Nobody dies from AIDS itself; instead they die from diseases like pneumonia, which are usually curable in people without AIDS.

AIDS is spread by a virus: HIV, the Human Immuno-deficiency Virus. It is this virus which attacks a person's immune system, causing them to become unable to fight off disease. Although it is deadly, HIV is a brittle virus, which means that unlike many other viruses, it cannot survive long outside the body. Because of this, it can only be passed from one person to another by means of exchanging bodily fluids like sperm or blood. Since blood for transfusions is now routinely screened to detect the presence of HIV, the only ways a person can normally get AIDS are through sharing equipment used in injecting drugs like heroin, or through having sex with an infected person.

One thing leads to another

Because HIV does not turn people lime green or make them grow an extra head, it can be very difficult to know who has it. Like most viruses, it is possible for people to carry HIV in their body for years before developing AIDS. So people can have HIV without even being aware of it.

And HIV does not discriminate. It will attack anyone. It doesn't matter if you're young or old, male or female, black or white, homosexual or heterosexual. It makes no difference if you've lived a life so bad that it would make Hitler blush or so good that it would make Mother Theresa green with envy. And it makes no difference whether you've had sex every day, twice a day, for umpteen years or are having it for the first time. The chances are exactly the same. If you have sex with someone who is carrying HIV, then you risk getting it yourself. And that eventually leads to AIDS.

Ouch!

Then there is the danger of getting sexually transmitted diseases (STDs) other than AIDS. In recent years, AIDS has hogged the headlines as far as STDs go, yet it is estimated that every year in the UK, hospitals treat about 500,000 new cases of other sexually transmitted diseases. These include herpes, syphilis, chancroid, gonorrhoea, genital chlamydia and pelvic inflammatory disease. For some of these there is no cure, and they can cause chronic ill health and, in some cases, even infertility.

And the risk of developing cervical cancer is now reckoned to be doubled in women who begin having sexual intercourse before the age of 17. The risk is also thought to be increased by having sex with a number of different partners.

It could be YOU!

Every year in the UK about 8,000 girls under the age of 16 have their lives turned upside down by becoming pregnant. Some do so deliberately: they want someone to love them unconditionally, or to need them. Perhaps they are looking for a sense of womanhood or independence from their family. Maybe they just want a baby so much they don't feel they can wait. The vast majority, however, become pregnant unintentionally.

Some women can try for years to get pregnant and never succeed. In the end, a number opt for artificial means of what is known as 'insemination'. Others can get pregnant without even trying . . . and even when they're deliberately trying *not* to.

In just the same kind of way, some men are more fertile than others. Being more fertile doesn't make you 'more of a man', just as being less fertile doesn't make you 'less of a woman': it's just the way things are. There are many reasons why some people are more or less fertile than others, and few of them are permanent. In men, it can be something as trivial as your choice in underwear! Because sperm is sensitive to temperature, getting sufficient ventilation around the testicles *can* make all the difference. So however sexy you might look in a posing pouch or skimpy briefs, if you eventually try for a baby, you might want to invest in some boxer shorts!

In other words, becoming pregnant is like a lottery: you never know whose number will come up next, so it pays not to take risks. Most unintentional pregnancies happen because people are uninformed or unprepared.

So what happens now?

There are no more profound consequences of sex than the creation of a human life. This is true whether a pregnancy is planned or accidental. But it is especially true when a woman gets pregnant without any thought for what life will be like for the child which results. Some serious thinking needs to take place.

For those who become pregnant unintentionally, there are basically three options:

- termination
- giving the child away for adoption
- keeping the child.

When choices run out

There are thousands upon thousands of abortions every year. Over one-third of all pregnant women between the ages of 15 and 19, and one-half of all pregnant young women between the ages of 13 and 15, end their pregnancy in abortion. In medical terms, this is called a 'termination'.

But, whatever the media might tell you, abortion is not like having a tooth out. Like all surgery, it carries risks. And it *can* have long-term consequences: feelings of loss, guilt and remorse, as well as physical side-effects such as internal bleeding or even, occasionally, becoming unable to get pregnant in the future.

Abortion is a hotly debated issue. Some people say that it's wrong; others insist that it's a woman's right to choose whether or not to have a child. But most people who have abortions do so because they feel that they have *no* choice. It is the only thing they think they *can* do. Perhaps they or their family cannot afford to bring up a child. Perhaps they lack the support they need from family and friends.

You need to make your choices carefully early on, because abortion is not so much a choice as a sign that your choices have run out.

So long, farewell

Most young women decide against a termination of their pregnancy. They feel that they want to or have to see it through until the birth. A number of these, however, choose to give the baby up for adoption shortly after the birth. Some do so because they can't afford to keep the child. Some don't want to miss out on work or education. Some feel that they are not yet ready to become a full-time mother. And some believe that other people would be better prepared and better able to give their child the love and support they feel it needs.

It can be heart-wrenching to give away a baby you have nurtured for nine months, whether you ideally wanted the child or not. Some young women find that they cannot in the end go through with the adoption proceedings. Those who do go through with them can suffer for years afterward from feelings of grief or remorse.

And it's not just the mother who can be affected by such a far-reaching decision. However loving their new, adoptive parents might be, most people who have been adopted are filled with questions: Why did my mother give me away? Was it my fault? Was there something wrong with me?

Some adopted people search for their birth parent(s) almost as soon as they are legally able, at the age of 18. (It is illegal for birth parents to make the first contact with their children.) Usually they have one question in mind: Why did you give me away?

For some, these are just questions. But for others, the questions can eat away at their self-esteem. They can be dogged by feelings of inadequacy. And however irrational these feelings might be, they will not go away.

The family way

Pregnancy can be a wonderful experience, but it can equally be painful and uncomfortable. The truth is, it's different for different people. Morning sickness, backache, food cravings, swollen legs, always having to sleep on your back, always needing the loo, always having to wear unfashionable clothes . . . pregnant women suffer in varying amounts from any or all of these.

With enough emotional and financial support from your family and friends, it can be a wonderful time. But if there's no one who understands your sudden desperate craving for a charcoal-and-chocolate pizza, life can be tough.

And raising a child is expensive. Even with emotional support, and with family members or close friends who are prepared to help out on the practical side, being a parent when resources are stretched can be very tough.

Having a child can be an extremely rewarding experience. But ask any parent and they will agree that it also requires enormous sacrifices. Your entire world revolves around a tiny person who just eats, sleeps, cries, turns a perfectly ordinary nappy into something which both looks and smells radioactive, and wakes you up in the middle of the night . . . *every* night!

However glad they are that they chose to keep their baby, teenage mothers often mourn the loss of their freedom and social life. It's as though the responsibility of having a baby robs you of being young.

'It takes two, baby!'

Getting pregnant doesn't just affect young women. So what about the fathers?

Although they can't, of course, get pregnant themselves, many young men are deeply shaken by the knowledge that they have made someone else pregnant. Some are delighted, others horrified. Some deny reality and act as though it had never happened, or else claim that someone else was the father. Others face up to their responsibilities.

Thirty years ago, if a boy got a girl pregnant, he was expected to marry her. These were known as 'shotgun' weddings, because it was imagined that if the boy was reluctant, the girl's father would march him up the aisle and make him 'an offer he couldn't refuse'!

Today, things are less clear. A guy who gets a girl pregnant outside marriage has no clear influence over what happens next, and his role is very far from defined. His options, or the options imposed on him, can include, for instance:

- total exclusion
- occasional access to the child
- finding a job to pay for its upkeep
- moving in with her parents
- marriage.

It can be a very traumatic and confusing time. And very few teenage fathers feel ready to take on the weighty responsibilities of parenthood.

'One small step for man, a giant leap for mankind'

But not all the harmful effects of sex with the wrong person or at the wrong time are physical. For lots of people, its emotional effects can prove just as hurtful.

If you're 'in love', sex can seem like the natural thing to do, the logical 'next step'. But it's a big step to take. Sex often heightens and complicates people's emotional involvement with their boyfriend or girlfriend. And if this is one-sided, or if the relationship is short-lived, it's bound to leave someone emotionally scarred. As a result, their self-esteem can hit rock bottom.

For lots of people, their first experience of sex is not planned. They just get carried away, or their boyfriend or girlfriend pushes them into it as 'proof' of their love. They end up with very mixed feelings about sex because they did not feel ready for it.

Sadly, there are many people who have felt used for

another person's pleasure. Their experience of sex is damaging because it took place in the wrong way, at the wrong time and often with the wrong person. It was meant to be a special experience, but actually it turned into something harmful and negative.

Sex is not a sport like football. It's not a sign of maturity like shaving or growing breasts. And it's not a proof of love like a ring or a Valentine card. It's about sharing who you are with another person on a very intimate level. And it should be chosen freely by both parties.

Unfortunately, this is often not the case. As well as people feeling pushed into having sex, an alarming number of people are forced into having sex against their will.

'Just our little secret . . .'

Sadly, sexual abuse and mistreatment are all too common.

Many women (and men) have suffered from rape or sexual assault. When rape happens to someone under the age of 16, it is known as 'child sexual abuse'. Sexual abuse can sometimes happen even to babies. It can happen to boys as well as girls. In most cases, a child is abused by someone they know and trust: a parent, a brother or sister, an uncle or aunt, a neighbour or a friend of the family.

It is usual for the person doing the abuse to insist that it remain a secret and that it's just their way of expressing love. It can range from touching a child's genitals to inserting a penis or some other object into the child's anus or vagina.

Although sexual abuse and rape involve sex, they really have more to do with power. People who rape or sexually abuse others are exerting power over their victims and taking away their choice. And worst of all, they usually make their victims feel that it was their own fault, even though there was actually nothing they could do to stop it.

People who have been raped or abused often feel dirty, guilty, worthless or unlovable because their most intimate form of expressing affection has been hijacked by someone else for their selfish pleasure.

Sex is meaningful only when you positively *choose* to do it. And for people who have suffered rape or abuse, it can be a long and painful journey to recover this feeling of choice.

If you've been the victim of sexual abuse, there is advice on what to do and where to get help in 'Taking Control', Chapter 13 of this book.

A ladder for the top shelf

Then there is pornography. Though some people would argue that pornography is 'just a bit of fun', it actually cheapens both women and men.

Pornography devalues people by turning them into objects rather than human beings. When men stand together in a huddle, their tongues hanging out, gawping at a full colour centre-page spread of a nude model, whatever it is that they find impressive, it's certainly not her personality!

Pornography works by stimulating people's sexual

desires, through either the written word or pictures. Women tend on the whole to be turned on more by atmosphere and imagination, evoked more easily by a piece of text than by pictures. Men, on the other hand, tend to react more to visual stimulation.

Of course, not all nude pictures or sex scenes in films and books are pornographic. Even the Bible contains an erotic and sexually explicit poem!

So what's the difference? Simply this: pornography is more concerned with the sex than with the person or story. And the danger is that people who use pornography also end up becoming more concerned with the sex than with who their partner is as a person.

Pornography makes sex into an item for sale. What becomes important is not the other person, but simply having your own desires met – getting what *you* want.

'I'm all tied up right now'

There is also the more 'bizarre' side of sex. Fetishes such as bondage, domination and sado-masochism are rarely healthy, despite what some people claim: they normally have to do with controlling someone's identity and behaviour rather than accepting them freely for who and what they are.

And at their most extreme, these fetishes can lead to damaging and dangerous pursuits such as 'auto-erotic asphyxiation'. Over the years, quite a few people have died doing this, including most famously one MP.

Fragile: handle with care

So, whilst everyone has sexual desires and drives, it is clear that not every expression of them is a good thing.

Whilst sex itself is a perfectly natural thing, we have to treat it with great care – in exactly the same way as anything else of great value.

We cannot indulge in it recklessly without suffering the consequences. We're not just flesh and bone: we're people with emotions and feelings.

So sex, because it is an act which intimately involves two people, cannot just be reduced to a physical activity like jogging. We instinctively know that it means more.

And the sexual decisions you make are not just personal: they can have important implications for others, families and the whole of society. It is important to think about how your decisions will affect others before you make them.

Questions

- Why do you think so many people assume that the negative consequences of sex, like AIDS or an unwanted pregnancy, will never happen to them?
- Do you think it's true that people's first experience of sex makes a big impression?
- What happens when love and sex get separated?

5

Accidents can happen

PICTURE THE SCENE. . . It's Friday night, your parents are out, you're alone in your room with your boyfriend or girl-friend. You shove some smoochy music on the stereo and soon you're in each other's arms . . . and throats . . . and trousers . . .

Now if we're honest, when we have the hots for someone, we know that there comes a point when our brains shut down and we find it very hard to control our desires. No matter how self-disciplined we are, we can easily forget it all when our hormones take over. Of course, we never *mean* for it to happen this way, but things just go too far . . .

As we saw in the last chapter, very few of the teenage girls who get pregnant each year plan for it. In fact, in a survey of pregnant teenagers done by the Family Planning Association, almost one-third of those asked said that they got pregnant simply because they 'got carried away' and didn't know how to stop.

There are two very simple ways to avoid unwanted pregnancies:

- using contraceptives
- not having sex.

The A—Z of contraception

There are about a dozen commonly recognised forms of contraception. There are disadvantages to all of them, though more with some than others. They fall roughly into three categories:

Permanent
This involves minor surgery, so it's not for the fainthearted or the indecisive – and definitely not for teenagers! In women, the Fallopian tubes connecting the ovaries to the womb are cut or blocked. This is sometimes called 'female sterilisation' or 'tubal ligation'. In men, the *vas deferens* connecting the testes to the penis are snipped; the operation is known as a 'vasectomy'. The estimated failure rate for both is approximately 0.1 per cent.

Long term
These are all for women, and include:
- the intra-uterine device (IUD), a T-shaped plastic and copper gadget inserted into the womb for five years;
- slow-release hormonal implants, slipped under the skin of the upper arm by a doctor and good for five years; and
- the injection of a slow-release hormone, good for two or three months, but not for the squeamish!
Each of these have a normal failure rate of around 1 per cent.

Short term

These are mainly also all for women, and include:

- the *Pill* (there are actually two different basic types), estimated to have a failure rate of less than 1 per cent if used carefully, but you have to remember to take them regularly;

- the *'natural method'* of counting days and recording body temperature and other signs that a woman is at her most fertile, avoiding sex at this time. This fails in anywhere between 2 and 20 per cent of cases, but has the distinction of being the only form of contraception fully endorsed and approved by the Roman Catholic Church;

- the *diaphragm*, a rubber cap shaped a bit like an old World War One army helmet, placed inside the vagina over the cervix and used with spermicide, with an estimated failure rate of between 4 and 18 per cent; and

- the *sponge*, a soft round sponge filled with spermicide which acts like a diaphragm but has a failure rate of between 10 and 25 per cent. Like the diaphragm, the sponge tends to cut down on the spontaneity of the occasion, since it needs to be inserted just prior to sex;

- *condoms*. There are both male and female condoms, thin sheaths of rubber which line the penis or vagina like thin, transparent rubber gloves, and collect sperm before it has a chance to enter the vagina itself. *This is the only form of contraception which can protect against HIV infection.* Condoms come in a range of colours, sizes (though men are more likely to buy condoms labelled 'humungous' than 'microscopic', whatever the actual size of their penis, which is why smaller condoms are often sold as being 'snug-fitting' or 'contoured'!), thicknesses and, for use in oral sex, even flavours! But although they are reckoned to be 98 per cent effective when used by adults, the Family Planning Association estimates that when used by teenagers, the failure rate can be as high as 15 per cent.

In addition to these, there is the so-called 'emergency Pill', which can be used up to three days after sexual intercourse to prevent the fertilised egg from attaching itself to the wall of the womb. It is roughly 96 per cent effective. Many doctors are worried that some women are using this as an alternative to regular contraception. They are not convinced that it is safe, since it was designed only for *emergency* use, and has not undergone the rigorous testing needed for *regular* use.

Withdrawing the penis during sex, before you ejaculate, really has no contraceptive value at all. The technical latin term for it is *'coitus interruptus'*, literally meaning 'interrupted sex'. It is said that during the Middle Ages, when adultery was considered a terrible sin (but still went on), wealthy men would sometimes instruct their servants to interrupt them when they were having it away with their mistresses, because it didn't technically count as adultery unless the man 'came'. They could therefore have their 'bit on the side' without any of the guilt!

Although the sperm ejaculated during sex will not go into the womb if the man withdraws before the end, the failure rate is between 20 and 25 per cent. This is not only because the timing is extremely difficult to get right, but also because small amounts of sperm-filled lubricant are emitted by the penis *before* a man reaches his orgasm, which could be enough to make a woman pregnant.

Contraceptives are designed to stop a woman getting pregnant. With the exception of condoms, which were designed specifically to stop the spread of sexually transmitted diseases, none of them give any protection whatsoever against HIV and AIDS.

And none of them, *including condoms*, are 100 per cent effective. Which is why sex with a condom is now know as 'safer' sex, not 'safe' sex.

So the only absolutely certain, tried and tested, positively guaranteed method of not getting pregnant is . . . don't have sex!

Prevention or cure?

As far as AIDS is concerned, since there is no cure, prevention is everything.

And just as there are two ways to avoid getting pregnant, there are two ways to prevent yourself from becoming 'HIV positive':
• always use a condom during sex; or
• do not have sex with anyone who might possibly have the virus.

But, of course, it is very hard to know who has been sleeping with whom. People often lie about their past misadventures, so it's very difficult to know who might have the virus, especially since it can take years to show itself. And the evidence so far is that the failure rate for condoms in preventing the spread of AIDS is the same as their failure rate in preventing pregnancy.

So the only sure-fire way of not getting AIDS is only ever to have sex with someone who only ever has sex with you (and has only ever had sex with you).

As the World Health Organisation puts it, 'the most effective way to prevent HIV transmission is to abstain from sexual intercourse or for two uninfected partners to remain faithful to one another. Otherwise the risk of spreading HIV can be significantly reduced by using condoms.'

Safe sex?

As we've seen, of course, physical things such as unwanted pregnancies or sexually transmitted diseases are not the only negative consequences that can come from having sex with the wrong people or at the wrong time.

And even if we accept the fact that none of the available contraceptives can give us 100 per cent protection against pregnancy and AIDS, all too often we forget that none of them can give *even the slightest protection* against the various different non-physical consequences of sex we've been examining.

Questions

- How much do you know about the various forms of contraception?
- How do they compare with one another?
- Do you think you would have the courage to insist on using a condom during sex?

6

Do the right thing

WE ALL KNOW that valuable things need to be looked after.

If you had a Rolls Royce or Ferrari, you wouldn't take it on a cross-country rally, or drive it off a cliff. You'd drive it the way it's supposed to be driven, polish it and keep it well maintained.

Likewise, you wouldn't wear your favourite jeans for painting the ceiling. Or use your best CD as a frisbee for the dog to fetch. To do so would be stupid – you'd spoil them.

But your sexuality is far more important than a car or your clothes. Because of this, you need to take care of it. The fact is that if you do not make your sexual choices carefully, you will damage something more valuable than anything else you have – yourself.

The dangers of double chocolate caramel crunch

Take ice cream, for example. Most of us love ice cream. But gorging on it is not just selfish, it can damage your appetite. In the end, if you were to spend all day, every day, stuffing yourself with raspberry ripple, not only would you be extremely unhealthy, you would slowly lose any pleasure you had in eating it. You might never want to look at a Häagen Dazs carton again!

Sex and ice cream are both good: so good that it's important to be careful how we use them. Because abusing them could not only damage our enjoyment of them, but also do serious damage to ourselves.

Going through the motions

Sex is more than just a biological act: it involves our emotions and our feelings. A human being is more than just a collection of bodily fluids. We have what is usually referred to as a spirit or soul – the thing which makes us who we are, with all of our particular characteristics, our likes and dislikes, our feelings and emotions. We are not just biological machines – inefficient robots.

This means that sex is always more than bonking: it's an act which unites two people. It is a moment when two people become one. If sex *were* just about bonking and having an orgasm, then we wouldn't feel hurt or upset if we've been used. But we do. Sex is about a lot more than a physical experience.

Sexual intercourse should be an act of giving yourself totally to another person. That means trusting them and caring for them. It means being committed to them. It should never be just a way of satisfying your own desires.

Sex is about *giving* rather than *taking*.

Sex is meant to be about a *relationship*. It's meant to be about *love*. When it's not, in the end it's always an empty experience.

Questions

- Apart from feasting on ice cream, what areas of life can you think of in which self-discipline is important?
- How can you tell the difference between lust and love? How do you know when 'this is the one'?
- Do you think the way the media generally portrays sex is more about giving or taking?

7

What's love got to do with it?

THE WORLD OF TELEVISION and films is unreal. Many TV programmes and movies portray sex mainly as a casual, biological act. Sometimes, the two people involved love each other for more than just a night, but more often than not, all they are really interested in is having a quick screw.

And what's more, TV and films often glamorise sex. According to the average Hollywood blockbuster, it's always guaranteed to be a wonderful, fulfilling, earth-shattering experience.

From ANYWHERE With Love

Bond entered the room. He was tall and handsome, with a cruel but tender smile. The beautiful girl sitting at the table looked up at him and fluttered her eyelashes. Crossing to her, he smiled, cruelly but tenderly.

'Hello,' she whispered, in a voice that could melt butter.

'The name's Bond,' said Bond, confidently. 'James Bond.'

He kissed her passionately.

'Take me,' she breathed, suddenly slipping out of all of her clothes. 'Oh James, be cruel but tender with me . . .'

James Bond is an entirely fake world. It's a world where, thirty seconds after meeting the girl, James is in bed with her. In Bond's world, sex is always wonderful and without any long-term consequences. James Bond has never heard of condoms or AIDS. The women who fall into his arms never have periods, or headaches, or moods, and change with every film.

Bond is always muscular and his women are always beautiful. No one is ever tired or tense. Bond never gets cramp in full flow or fails to perform, and the women always have fully vocal, earth-moving multiple orgasms.

What does it matter, you might ask. After all, this is the movies, this is fantasy land . . .

Well, the problem is that many of us actually end up believing it can be true. Lots of people believe that, at least where sex is concerned, real life is exactly like the movies.

The fact is that James Bond and virtually all these movie sex scenes sell you a soft-focused, fully orchestrated, 'Surround Sound' . . . lie.

'Not now, darling, I have a headache'

The truth is that sex is often a wonderful experience. But it can equally be . . . well . . . messy.

Sheets are cold, people often aren't in the mood. Hair

48

gets in the way. The phone goes at the wrong moment. One of you is too tired. Or has eaten too much.

It can be very tender and romantic, but it can also be very ordinary, disappointing, mundane, humiliating, ungratifying, unfulfilling, uncomfortable . . . at times even boring.

Round the back of the bike sheds, having sex, you think that the earth will move. But you soon discover that the only things that do move are the bikes as they fall on top of you!

Making love, you see, takes practice, patience and commitment. Sometimes one partner will be more in the mood than the other. And men and women often enjoy different things about sex, and bring with them different expectations. Whilst men nearly always achieve orgasm, that's not true of women. Which can leave both of them feeling like they have somehow failed.

'Dedication — that's what you need'

To be enjoyed at its best, sex needs to take place within the context of a long-term, committed and permanent loving relationship. It can be good with someone you care about; but only in the security of a committed and permanent relationship can sex ever really be enjoyed at its best. It needs two people who love and trust each other enough not to worry when it goes wrong. It needs two people who are prepared to learn about each other and what brings pleasure to the other person.

But it's not just practice that makes sex satisfying: it needs to be with someone you love. And not only love, but also trust and respect.

Sex is about sharing yourself intimately with another person. The more shallow the relationship between partners, the more shallow the sex will be. The deeper the relationship, the more meaningful the sex.

That kind of sharing makes you vulnerable. To share yourself that deeply with someone, you need to be sure that they will not take the opportunity to hurt you. You need to trust them and know that they respect you. And in turn you need to earn their trust and respect them.

Hollywood wives — and husbands

When asked who was the greatest lover in Hollywood, one star replied that it was not promiscuity which made a lover great, but the ability to love one person well for forty-odd years. 'Anyone can sleep around,' they added. 'Even dogs do that!'

That's why, throughout history, people have discovered that the best place for sex is within a long-term, committed, loving relationship.

However you disguise it, we are talking marriage.

Questions

- Why do you think TV and the movies rarely show sex that isn't perfect?
- What makes sex in a long-term, committed relationship different from casual sex?
- Do you agree that sex is best within a permanent loving relationship? If so, why do you think so many people settle for second best?

8

'Married . . . with children'

THROUGHOUT HISTORY, the civilised world has always had, as part of its system, the idea of committed, permanent relationships. This idea has come down to us as marriage.

Marriage is not a modern thing. Nor is it a European or even a Christian thing. The ancient Greeks had marriages; so did the ancient Egyptians. The Romans believed in marriage, as did the Assyrians, the Babylonians, the Huns, the Goths, the Visigoths, the Barbarians, and all those other people who inhabited the ancient world. Not to mention people in Africa, Asia and America.

Even in our own time, every major society or country has its own codes about relationships and they all include the idea of marriage – that is, a permanent, committed relationship between two people.

Down . . . but not out

Why should this be? After all, marriage has a pretty bad press. More than one-third of all marriages in the UK end in divorce. And a number of those which remain intact still fail to rate very highly on the 'eternal bliss' stakes. Somewhere along the line, love and romance turn into habit and toleration.

For every marriage we know that works, most of us can think of one or two that haven't worked.

Yet if marriage were really so bad, or designed to spoil our fun as it often seems, then why should we see it cropping up consistently throughout human history? Surely someone, at some point, would have said, 'This is stupid', and come up with something better?

For instance: what about a non-renewable, fixed-term contract for three years, complete with shared use of living quarters, equal choice of television programmes, agreed division of the household chores, comprehensive three-times weekly bedroom rights, and a built-in opt-out clause for either side after 18 months? Why has something like this not caught on?

Perhaps the truth is that there *is* no better system than marriage. Perhaps we just have to try harder, or choose better. Or both. Maybe marriage, with all its faults and difficulties, has a lot more going for it than we've been led to believe. Maybe it really *is* the way in which humans were – and are – best suited to live together.

The interesting thing is that, within all the cultures which have marriage, two beliefs about it are common:
• it is the best environment for sex to take place;
• it is the best environment in which to bring up children.

'Love and marriage, love and marriage . . .'

Most cultures, whatever their religious background, have historically had laws forbidding people to have sex outside of marriage. In some, the punishment for committing adultery was very harsh indeed. In fact, adultery sometimes even carried the death penalty: a big price tag for a few moments of pleasure!

All that seems pretty steep today, given the ease with which people jump in and out of bed with each other, married or not.

Yet however tough, and even unjust, these punishments seem to us, their aim was simple: to keep sex within marriage. Why? Well, as we saw above, sex is best within the safety and security of a permanent, caring relationship. That's where we can get the most out of it. It's where children will generally grow up the most secure, and it's therefore what will safeguard the future health of society itself.

What's the big deal?

What's so special about marriage?

In our culture today, marriage is increasingly unpopular. As far as many people are concerned, it's old-fashioned: an out-of-date hangover from the past. As a result, fewer couples are getting married, and more and more are simply choosing to live together.

'After all,' they say, 'marriage is only a piece of paper, isn't it?'

Well . . . no. The truth is that the piece of paper – the marriage certificate – is nothing more than a symbol: it's a sign of everything else that marriage is about.

Marriage is actually about a lot more than just a nice ceremony, a white dress, aunties you haven't seen in twenty years (and don't really want to see for another twenty), cake, endless photographs, boring speeches, the worst hats you've ever seen in your life, and 26 toasters. *That's* a wedding!

The Beginner's Guide to Marriage

So what is marriage about? Well, it's about a lot of things, but four come particularly to mind.

Friendship
The first thing is friendship. Husbands and wives are friends and companions to each other. They love one another, which is, perhaps, the highest form of friendship. Your husband or wife should be your best friend – someone with whom you can discuss all your problems and share both the good times and the bad times. Your husband or wife should be someone who knows you intimately, your good points and your bad points, and who loves you for exactly who you are without reserve.

Support

A friend does more than just spend time with you and listen to you talk: they support you. In other words, you know that you don't have to be on top form all the time. Because when things go wrong and times are a little on the rough side, friends are there to pick you up – or at least to be there with you.

A husband or wife gives this kind of support; but marriage is about something extra. When you marry someone, you promise in front of your family and friends to love and support them for ever.

So with a marriage, you know that you have a partner who has committed themselves legally to giving you the support you need for as long as both of you are alive. Everybody goes through tough times, when they feel depressed or down, like not carrying on. But in marriage you know that your partner has promised to offer you the support and encouragement you need. That means you don't have to rely just on your own strength any more.

Family life

Marriage creates the best environment for family life. Of course, single or 'lone' parent families prove that families don't have to be 'Mum, Dad and the Kids'. In fact, many lone parents bring up their children with more love and security than other more 'traditional' families. Yet most people still agree that the *ideal* situation is to have children brought up in a secure, stable environment with both the mother and the father present.

Commitment

Perhaps most importantly, marriage is about making a promise – a public commitment to one person. A marriage vow is a statement that you will stick with your partner, no matter what happens. In a wedding service, the bride and groom promise to remain together 'till death us do part'.

Instinctively we want – perhaps need – the security of someone who loves us no matter what. We want someone we love to make an exclusive and permanent choice to love us and stick with us no matter what the future holds.

But in this day and age, promises appear to mean less and less. Politicians break their promises the moment they are elected. Manufacturers have to be forced by law to fulfil the claims they make for their products. Promises are easy to make: and, it seems, easy to break. Sadly, marriages break up with increasing frequency. Marriage has become virtually as disposable as a McDonalds wrapper or a soggy nappy.

In spite of this fact, every year thousands of couples tie the knot, in full knowledge of the fact that statistically they stand a one in three chance of ending the marriage in court rather than at the crematorium. These are not good odds. Perhaps that's why a lot of people choose just to live together. After all, you can't break a promise you haven't made. It's not that they don't love each other: they just don't feel able to make life-long promises.

But this turns *Mr* or *Ms Right* into *Mr* or *Ms Right For Now*. It's hardly very flattering. Or secure. Or confidence-building. 'Well *of course* I love you, darling. Very much. At least for the moment . . . or until someone better comes along.'

We live in a society in which, if you get fed up with something, you trade it in for a new one. But to do that with people is to treat them like objects. Marriage, with its promise to remain true to the other person no matter what, is treating them like a human being. It means not part-exchanging your old husband or wife for a new one, no matter how appealing the new model might be!

A former winner of the Nobel Peace Prize was once interviewed for television. In his 80s, he had been married for more than fifty years. When the interviewer asked him if he thought his wife was the most beautiful woman he knew, he replied, 'Of course not. She's 80! But she is the woman I love the most. She is the one I'm committed to.'

Marriage is about putting your money where your mouth is. It is legally binding. It's about making a *public* and *permanent* commitment. And in a constantly changing world, it's the quality and content of our commitments which define who we are.

More than meets the eye

All of this gives us a clue why it is important that sex should take place within marriage. Sex is a physical act which sums up all the other aspects of marriage. Sex should be about love and security.

Everybody is looking for love. But a lot of people settle

just for sex or romance, and are left feeling empty and cheated and bitter. When you're attracted to someone, it can be difficult to tell the difference between love and simple infatuation. And by the time you work out that this is not 'the one', it can be difficult to give up what you have, even if you know that it's ultimately doomed.

There's a lot more to marriage than just going to bed with one another. Marriages that are based purely on sexual attraction don't last long. When someone else comes along whom one of them is attracted to sexually, there's really nothing to keep husband and wife together. And that's only if the traditional argument about which end of the toothpaste tube you should squeeze from doesn't get them to the divorce courts first!

The fact is that for any relationship to work, it has to be based on security and trust. And this can only be assured by mutual commitment to one another – a promise to remain faithful.

That is why sex is at its best and most fulfilling within marriage. Because *sex is about more than itself*. It's both a physical and emotional experience. It's about the *people* who have sex, and the way they feel about each other, rather than the act itself.

The way sex is often portrayed in books and in the media makes you think that it's all about humping and bumping. It's almost as if memorising the *Kama Sutra* page by page, and training for Olympic Gold in gymnastics, is the way to achieve a truly fulfilling sex life.

But what really makes sex fulfilling is not technique. It's

not fitness. It's not size or strength. It's not even beauty. It's the people who have sex, and the relationship they have with one another. It's sharing who you are totally and intimately with another person.

So the ever-popular question, 'But don't we need to find out if we're sexually compatible before we get married?' misses the point. Because if you're compatible in other ways, you'll be compatible sexually. And if you're not compatible in other ways, no matter how good the sex may be at a technical level, it will never be enough.

Sex is at its best with someone you love, trust, support and have committed yourself to permanently. It's a way of showing them this love, trust, support and commitment. And it's also a lot of fun.

So if this is sex at its best, why settle for less?

Questions

- What makes marriage different from just living together?
- When you think about marriage, do you find yourself thinking more of a fairytale . . . or a nightmare?
- Are the qualities you look for when thinking about a future marriage partner the same as those you look for when you're deciding whether or not to go out with someone?

9
How not to go all the way

IF IT'S TRUE THAT sexual intercourse is best experienced as part of a long-term, committed marriage relationship, then it follows that we have to be careful how we handle sex before we enter into such a relationship. So the big question is, 'How far should I go sexually before marriage?' The truth is, there's no easy answer to this one.

It would be really handy to have a check list. You know, something along the lines of:
- 'you can kiss, but don't use your tongue';
- 'you can grope, but not to orgasm'; or
- 'you can fondle breasts, but don't undress'.

Unfortunately, it's not as simple as that.

Close to the edge

So how far should I go?

There is a story of a rich old woman who lived in a fabulous mansion halfway up a steep mountain. The only access was via a narrow and winding road. When her old chauffeur died, she interviewed drivers to take his place. She asked each of them just one question: 'How close to the edge could you take me without plunging down the mountain?'

The first replied, 'I could take you within two feet, but I wouldn't risk it further out than that.'

The second said, 'I'm so good, I could take you to within six inches of the edge.'

The third was more cautious: 'I wouldn't take you anywhere near the edge, madam. I don't believe in taking unnecessary risks.'

And who got the job? Number three.

It's the same way with relationships: it makes sense not to go too 'close to the edge'.

For example, many couples engage in what's technically known as 'heavy petting'. This is not wrestling with a St Bernard: it's groping around on a sofa with your clothes half off, fondling each other's boobs or balls.

It can include oral sex – otherwise known as a 'blow job' – where one person licks the other's penis or clitoris to orgasm.

When you've got this far, it's very easy to lose control altogether, 'get carried away' and end up having full vaginal sex. (In fact, it is pretty rare not to!) It makes sense, therefore, to draw a line further back, at a point where you are still in control.

'Let's talk about sex'

Ultimately, the only person who can set your limits is you. It's very important to think things through, and to set your own personal limits before you ever get into a relation-ship.

It's also essential to talk through with your boyfriend or girlfriend what you consider to be acceptable limits for the physical side of your relationship. This might send both of you a bright shade of purple with embarrassment, of course, but it's important to do it anyway.

You might feel that it's a good idea not to take off each other's clothes. Or not to touch the other person's genitals. The important thing is that you actually discuss it togeth-er. If one of you has more conservative limits than the other, then these are the limits which should be observed.

It is wrong to force someone into doing something they don't feel ready for. It is wrong to put undue pressure on them simply because it's what *you* want to do.

Arguments such as the ever-popular, 'If you really loved me, you'd do this', are nothing but emotional blackmail. If someone really loves you, they will respect your limits and will not try to make you do anything you don't feel entirely comfortable with. If they don't respect your lim-its, then they don't respect you. And if they don't respect you, they don't love you.

Your most important sexual asset

Agree your limits together. And avoid situations in which these limits will be tested beyond endurance. Because we are shy about this sort of thing, most of us never talk about what we see as acceptable, or desirable, and therefore set no limits. But it's obvious that, with no guidelines at all, you are that much more likely to lose control. It's perfectly natural to want to get physical with each other; but we must realise that, where the physical side of the relationship is concerned, things can easily get out of control.

Be sensible and mature. Know yourself, know your partner, set your limits and take precautions. Think! You might have made the mistake of assuming that your face, or eyes, or hair, or legs, or chest, or backside, or vagina, or penis, is your greatest sexual asset. If you have, think again. The truth is that your most important sex organ is your brain. So *use it!*

We all occasionally make mistakes, but with enough care we can ensure that we don't go over the edge.

The only thing in the world?

After all, there's more to life than sex.

So try to develop interests together, to be good company for each other, building an all-round friendship. Don't spend all your time locked in a room playing tonsil hockey.

Because any relationship that is going to last has to be based on more than physical attraction.

It sounds strange at first, but in terms of secure and lasting relationships, the truth is that 'beauty' is probably the least important aspect! Of course, it may initially attract us to the other person, but its fascination will eventually wear thin. To prove the point, men with beautiful wives still have affairs, even when their lover is much less attractive than their wife. Beauty and novelty are often mistaken for one another.

We have all known people who got into relationships based purely on physical attraction. Sometimes these relationships worked out, but only when the couple discovered things in common. Far more often they failed. Because after they had spent a few days or weeks admiring each other, and perhaps even got over the initial novelty of bonking each other, these people discovered that they actually had nothing to say to one another.

Bimbos and Himbos have a very limited shelf life! Because no matter how good-looking you may be, what is *really* attractive to people is who you are as a person.

Questions

- What limits would you set in a relationship, and why?
- How would you get over the embarrassment of talking about your limits with a boyfriend or girlfriend?
- Besides sexual attraction, what is it that appeals to you about the people you fancy?

10

Young, free and single

BUT WHAT IF YOU haven't actually got a boyfriend or girl-friend?

Women's and men's magazines are crammed full of articles on:
- how to get your man or woman;
- how to make yourself irresistible;
- how to make yourself huggable;
- what to do with your partner once you've got them;
- how to satisfy them in bed;
- what they most want sexually . . .

The list is endless.

The entire point of existence, it seems, is to get and keep your woman or man. Not having a boyfriend or girlfriend is not good for the image: it can make you feel inferior. After all, 'real men' have no difficulty in attracting women, and 'attractive women' have no trouble getting a man. If only you were like them . . .

It seems as though having a boyfriend or girlfriend is the way to prove you're a success: it's a status symbol. And if you don't have a partner, then there must be something wrong with you. You must be a failure. You must be weak, or ugly, or both.

Faced with such pressures, the temptation is to get off with the first available person that doesn't look like The Creature from the Black Lagoon. After all, we don't want to be a failure. And if we have a boyfriend or girlfriend – any boyfriend or girlfriend – then surely that means that we are a success.

But is it really true that we need to be in a relationship with someone to be 'whole'? Let's take a look at some of the myths.

'Who's gonna love you when you're old and fat and ugly?'

Myth No. 1: *'Having a partner proves I'm attractive.'*

It's estimated that around 85 per cent of teenagers don't like the way they look. Their nose is too big. Their teeth are crooked. Their ears stick out. They're covered in zits. Their hair is the wrong colour. They're too fat, or their bum's the wrong shape, or their boobs are too big, or too small, or their stomach sticks out, or their legs are too fat, or too short, or too skinny, or their beard won't grow, or stop growing, or . . . well, you get the idea. But who are they comparing themselves with?

Not many of us are built like super-models. Nor is there any reason why we should be. But because the media, TV and magazines are filled with beautiful, perfectly formed, size 10 women and muscle-bound, bronzed, handsome men, we fall into the trap of thinking that this is the norm – the way we should be. If only we were 'attractive', we think, *then* we would be happy . . .

But it's important that we recognise three things:

- *Supermodels don't really look like their photographs.* Without the two-hour make-up sessions, the expert lighting, the expensive clothes, the flamboyant hairstylists, the exotic locations, the personal trainers, the professional photographers, and the 267 lousy shots taken just to get one good one (which is often touched up afterwards, anyway, to remove any 'blemishes'), even supermodels look kind of . . . well . . . ordinary. Those who work in the fashion industry know that they are selling a fantasy, but half the time the rest of us believe it to be real.

- *Even people we think of as stunningly attractive are rarely happy with the way they look.* We might think that film and pop stars are attractive, but they don't necessarily agree. In fact, many of them end up spending a fortune trying to improve their looks, fuelling tabloid debates as to how much of them is real and how much is plastic.

- *Being attractive does not necessarily bring happiness.* Even if you do look like a super-model, it doesn't guarantee that you will have any more 'success' in relationships than the rest of us. Princess Diana is considered beautiful the world over, but it's no secret that her marriage has failed. And Hollywood stars are even worse. In the 1950s, Elizabeth Taylor was one of the most beautiful women in the world, yet she's been married eight times (at last count). Marilyn Monroe must have been one of the most attractive women who ever lived. Her string of boyfriends even included US President John Kennedy. Yet she died lonely and scared, divorced from her third husband, taking her own life through an overdose of sleeping tablets (conspiracy theories aside). She just couldn't face living any more. She was only 36.

The idea that being 'attractive' brings happiness is simply wrong. The fact is that being 'attractive' is not just about what we look like. It is about *who we are* – our thoughts, our interests, our attitudes . . . in fact, everything that makes us *us!*

And anyway, even good looks are a matter of personal judgment rather than objective fact. Beauty, as they say, is in the eye of the beholder.

'The man who has everything'

Myth No. 2: *'Having a partner proves I'm successful.'*

We all know how to recognise a successful business person. They make deals on their mobile phone. They drive a Mercedes, a Porsche or a BMW. They wear a gold Rolex watch and an expensive suit. The things they own are status symbols – displaying to the world that they are (sound the trumpets) . . . *successful.*

But sometimes this kind of person extends the idea of status symbols even to their relationships. They choose people as their partners who will make them look good. Like the power-dressed woman business executive who parades her toyboy in front of her friends or colleagues. Or the middle-aged businessman with an expensively dressed young blonde on his arm, less than half his age. 'Look at me,' he's saying. 'I have everything – a Porsche, a penthouse and a beautiful woman.'

Although we don't necessarily want the same status symbols as the successful business person, it's easy to get trapped into thinking the same way. 'If only I had someone to go out with,' we think, '*then* I'd be a success. It would prove I'm worth something.'

When you think about it, this is a pretty stupid idea. Success doesn't lie in any of these things. And some of the most 'successful' people have also been some of the most unhappy.

Elvis was the most successful singer the world has ever known, married to a very beautiful woman. Yet he died of a drug overdose, like Marilyn a deeply unhappy person. And Kurt Cobain, lead singer with Nirvana, put a bullet through his head in spite of his fame, his marriage and his child.

'I can't get no satisfaction'

Myth No. 3: '*Having a partner will make me fulfilled.*'

Being in a stable, loving relationship is a very fulfilling experience. But that doesn't mean that you can only be fulfilled by going out with someone. Humans find fulfilment in many things: their job, their hobbies, their achievements, their interests, their friends, their faith.

Mother Theresa has spent her life helping the poor in the slums of Calcutta. By anyone's standards she's an extremely successful, fulfilled woman. Yet she doesn't have a partner. (It's against the rules for a nun!)

The idea that, if you are not in a relationship, you are somehow unfulfilled or unhappy, simply is not true. There are many thousands of people who are quite happy to be 'young, free and single'. Or even old, free and single. And thousands more who regret that they pinned their hopes of fulfilment on a relationship.

Periods of loneliness and feelings of isolation are a part of life, and occur in the best of marriages as well as amongst single people. It is quite possible to be in an ideal marriage and still be unfulfilled. Because fulfilment is never found in just one thing. Human life is complex, and true fulfilment is only ever found in a combination of things.

Fit bodies, fat minds

So if you are not in a relationship, don't worry. Don't allow yourself to get too intense about all this. Don't let it take over your life.

And don't spend your time searching for someone with the brains of Albert Einstein and the looks of Marilyn

Monroe or Arnold Schwarzeneggar in the hope that they will give you what you feel you're missing. You're in danger of ending up with someone with the brains of Marilyn Monroe or Arnold Schwarzeneggar and the looks of Albert Einstein! And you'll still feel that you're missing something.

Instead, use your time wisely. Use it to learn new skills and develop a wide range of interests. Broaden your appeal to other people by becoming a more interesting and more fulfilled person.

The person at school who has no problems finding boyfriends or girlfriends, and who spends their time groping and bonking their way to popularity with the opposite sex (and, especially in the case of girls, often unpopularity with their own), can too easily end up becoming twice-divorced and unsatisfied by the time they're 30.

Those who spend more time at school and at home developing their interests are more likely to turn 30 with a sense of achievement and fulfilment.

In the long run, *interesting* people are more attractive than physically beautiful ones. Especially when middle age sets in and, whoever you are, your assets head south and you begin to sag.

Above all, avoid pinning your sense of self-worth simply on your attraction to the opposite sex and your 'success' in relationships.

Questions

- What makes a good relationship? What makes a bad one?
- What do you look for in a boyfriend or girlfriend?
- Why do you think being single is not thought highly of in our society?

11

Behind closed doors

LET'S TALK about masturbation.

Masturbation is solo sex, what Woody Allen called 'Sex with someone you love'! It is the technical term for what is commonly known as 'wanking': stimulating your penis or clitoris, usually until you reach a climax.

It's different from a 'wet dream', because it requires some direct, 'hands on' action. It also requires you to be conscious! 'Wet dreams' can only occur when you are asleep. In other words, they're out of your control. And in spite of their name, you don't even need to have been dreaming about sex to have one. In men, they are the result of an involuntary erection, when sperm seeps out of the penis. There is a direct equivalent in women, called a 'nocturnal orgasm', in which fluid seeps out of the vagina.

For some reason masturbation is one of those things that rarely gets discussed, although it's the subject of volumes of toilet-wall poetry. As a result, people can end up believing that it's some kind of terrible perversion, and that no one else in the world does it, or has ever done it, except them. Which means they must be a freak.

Wrong.

The Big 'M'

A recent survey showed that approximately 95 per cent of all single men masturbate. (And the other 5 per cent were probably lying when they filled in the form!) Nor is it just 'a male thing' – something like 60 per cent of single women masturbate at one time or another. Even lots of married people masturbate.

Many of these people feel guilty about it.

People can start masturbating as young as 11 or 12. And although it's more common in young people than in older people, there's no top age limit for masturbation. You can keep on doing it till the day you die.

So it's pretty odd, when you think about it, that calling someone a 'wanker' should be considered an insult. After all, a lot of the time it's merely stating the obvious.

Time to start learning braille?

There are a lot of old wives' tales about masturbation. The most common one is that it will make you go blind. The most bizarre is that it causes hair to grow on the palms of your hands. The Victorians even believed that men could die as a result of what they discreetly termed 'solitary vices'. But the reality is that there is no evidence whatsoever that masturbation harms you physically in any way.

Of course, just because something doesn't harm you physically, that doesn't mean that it's necessarily an unreservedly good thing to get into the habit of doing, or that you are missing out if you're *not* doing it. Simply because you won't need a new pair of prescription specs, or permanently take to wearing gloves in public, this doesn't mean that you should lock yourself in your bedroom with an industrial size box of Kleenex and go all out for a new world record!

This chapter is written to help you understand masturbation, and to take away any irrational worries you might have about it. It's *not* meant as a Beginner's Guide.

So if you don't masturbate, it doesn't mean that you're weird. And there's no reason why you should start experimenting with it now.

Although there are no medical side-effects to masturbation, there are nevertheless several important things to think about. Because in solo sex, just as in sex with a partner, there are some possible emotional consequences to consider.

Out of control

Masturbation can be addictive. And any habit which enslaves you, which begins to control you, is harmful to you. It could be drugs like nicotine or cocaine. It could be alcohol. Gambling. Shopping. Video games. It could even be football or tiddleywinks. We can become addicted to all sorts of things. And even if they are good in themselves, if they reach the point where they control us rather than us controlling them, we should avoid them.

Sexual desires and urges can be very strong indeed. And the advantage of masturbation is that you don't need anyone else to satisfy them. Given a spare five minutes, and a little privacy, masturbation can be done virtually anywhere at any time.

But any urge that easy to satisfy can be habit-forming. And masturbation tends to be a very habit-forming activity. The more ingrained a habit becomes, the more difficult it is to break. And that's where it can become an addiction.

If masturbation controls us – and like all sexual urges, it easily can – then it is definitely harmful. Not because it is masturbation, but because it is an obsession.

Let your fingers do the walking

Masturbation can affect the way we think: and what we think affects us just as much as what we do.

Masturbation usually requires an element of sexual fantasy. It is rare for the physical sensations alone to be able to bring a person to climax, which is generally the goal of masturbation. And it is even more rare for a person to find sufficient erotic stimulation from the train timetable or the *Yellow Pages*.

Whilst most people who masturbate rely on mental pictures from their memories and imaginations to bring them off, some need visual stimulation. Often this means pornography. And the danger of all this is that, as we've already said, it encourages people to think of others as sexual objects rather than as full human beings. We stop thinking of them as *people* and reduce them to impersonal objects for our own sexual gratification, in order to reach an orgasm.

In addition, it's possible for people to become so used to 'coming' through masturbation that they find later on – when they *do* have a sexual partner – that the enjoyment they're able to receive from other types of stimulation is limited, leading to problems in the relationship.

The world-famous solo double act

Masturbation is an incomplete act.

Sex is about communication. Ideally, it's about making yourself 'one' with someone you love and trust. It's about the person you have sex with, not the sex itself.

Masturbation is sex with yourself, without a relationship, communication or intimacy. So ultimately, masturbation is not the real thing. It is incomplete. It's a double act with only one player. Because of this, if people masturbate a lot, they can end up with a sense of incompleteness, loneliness or even boredom from the experience, rather than the mixture of pleasure or guilt they initially felt.

Often this can lead people to look for bigger sexual thrills in full-blown sex. Not so much because they are in love as because they are bored and unsatisfied by the sense of incompletion left after masturbating.

This doesn't mean that we should rush out and experience the real thing. But it is true that for many people masturbation stops, or at least greatly reduces, after marriage. It's no longer necessary. Within marriage, we can experience sex as it should be, at its best.

If you are worried that masturbation has become a real problem for you, then get advice from an older person you trust.

But whatever you do, don't think that you are the only person ever to masturbate. Masturbation is a common experience for both men and women.

Questions

- Why don't people talk about masturbation?
- Why do you think that so many people feel guilty about masturbating?
- Do you think we are ever really honest about anything to do with our sexuality?

12

What if it's gone wrong?

ENDING RELATIONSHIPS can be painful.

Most of the terms that get used to describe the ending of a relationship reflect the various distorted ideas we have talked about throughout this book. People get 'dropped', 'dumped' or 'chucked' – as if what we were talking about was a discarded piece of rubbish – an object rather than a living, breathing human being.

If you feel that you have been treated as an object, as a thing, then try to remember the simple truth that *you are valuable for who you are, not who you date*. As we've seen, our value as people does not stem from our relationships with the opposite sex.

Out of the frying pan, into the fire

But here comes a piece of very important advice: however you feel, *if your relationship has broken up, resist the temptation to rush straight into another one*. Relationships formed on the 'rebound' often stem more from the need to find a 'replacement', to fill the gap in your life and to take away the loneliness, than from a genuine desire to be with the other person. And this means that you yourself are treating someone else like an object.

Wait until you are less vulnerable. Spend time with your friends. Develop your interests and hobbies. If you do form another relationship, wait until you can be sure that you're going out with someone because you like *them*, not simply the fact of having a boyfriend or girlfriend.

Remember that just because you are not going out with someone does not mean that you are unattractive, unsuccessful or unfulfilled. The world around you may try to pressurise you into forming relationships by making you feel a failure if you are 'unattached'. But the truth is that it is perfectly possible for you to be a totally fulfilled human being and at the same time young, free and single.

'Dear John . . .'

What if you are the person ending the relationship? Let's be honest: this is a task which is never easy. But having said that, there are things you can do which will help or hinder what eventually has to be. So what are they?

First, if you're going out with someone and you know that they are the wrong person for you, don't keep them hanging on. Honesty requires a great deal of courage, but it's better than deceit.

It is important when breaking up with someone, especially if they still like you a lot, to explain *why* you are breaking up with them, and to let them know where they stand. Beating about the bush may be easier in the short term, but it will actually result in all sorts of problems as time goes by, and leave your 'ex' more hurt than ever.

But it's also important to be sensitive. Being clear, firm and honest is one thing, but there are ways *to* and ways *not to* tell people things.

It may well be honest to tell someone straight up that their breath smells worse than the local rubbish tip, or that their new outfit makes them look like Mr Bean. But there are more tactful and constructive ways of saying the same thing. People usually reject criticism of themselves because it sounds like an attack, not because it's wrong.

When you're breaking up with someone, it's vital that you tell them what's *right* with them – what they've got going for them – not merely why they're not right for you. Be truthful. Think hard about what their good qualities are. But don't be patronising. They may well be hurting, but they are not objects for your pity.

Above all, when you break up with someone, give them a chance to speak. Listen carefully to what they have to say about themselves, you and your relationship. When relationships break up, the fault is never entirely one sided. Even though the relationship may be over, there are always things you can learn from it about yourself for the future.

Remember that it is important, if you have hurt someone, to ask for their forgiveness; and if necessary, to make amends as far as you can. And since, when we hurt someone else, we often also hurt ourselves, it is important also to learn to forgive yourself.

A new beginning

If you've gone further than you intended, and made a mistake sexually, it's not the end of the world. You can begin again.

Of course, mistakes have consequences. And obviously, the more serious the mistake, the more serious the consequences may prove to be. But the important thing is that, instead of just worrying about things and getting your problems out of perspective, you learn from your experience and find help if you need it.

If you've had sex, and think you may have contracted a disease or become pregnant, then you should seek help from your GP or another doctor. Remember that they are qualified to give you the best help possible, and their advice will be in strict confidence. You can trust them.

If you've had sex and feel used or disappointed, or even guilty, then you might want to talk to an older person whom you trust. It can be very helpful to talk things through with someone who is wiser and has more experience of life than you.

Some suggestions about people you can talk to, in confidence and without fear that they will judge you, are given at the end of this book.

Although we all have to accept the emotional, social or physical consequences of our mistakes, they should never become a trap from which we can't escape. You *can* change your behaviour. You *can* move on. You *can* start again. It's not the end – it can be a new beginning.

Questions

- Why do you think some people rush straight into another relationship when one has ended?
- How often do you think people drag emotional baggage into one relationship which was not solved in the last one? How much of a problem is it?
- Can you think of anyone who has made mistakes in life and yet has recovered from them?

13

Taking control

YOUR BODY BELONGS to you. No one else. But sometimes we feel pressured into doing all sorts of things that, with hindsight, we would rather not have done, and nowhere is this more true than when it comes to sex. It's all too easy to be pushed into believing that you are nobody unless you have 'done it', and that saying 'No' to somebody will stop them from liking you. And we all want to be liked. That's why comments such as, 'If you love me, you'll have sex with me', can be such powerful arm-twisters.

Your body, however, is part of you. Your sexuality is a valuable gift, not some cheap toy which you should allow anyone else to play around with.

'I can resist everything except temptation'

If you've never had sex with anyone, you should understand that virginity is not a stigma, but a healthy lifestyle choice. You can only give it away once, so make sure that you are in full control of the time, the place and the person you choose to give it away to.

It often calls for tremendous courage to resist someone who wants to have sex with you. What's even harder is when you *want* to have sex with them, and yet at the same time *don't* want to have sex with them. It's all very confusing. Your hormones say yes, but your brain cells say no. And actually saying no when your body is telling you to say yes can be very difficult indeed.

If it's hard at the best of times, if either of you has been drinking alcohol it can be almost impossible. The more you drink, the more your inhibitions disappear, and you find yourself doing things you would never dream of doing when you're sober, and usually regretting them the next morning.

Sometimes you would like to have sex with someone *eventually*, but don't feel ready at the moment. Or want to wait until marriage. Even so, it is extremely hard to resist someone when you fancy them like crazy and really care about them. And the more you care, the more difficult it becomes.

But the strange thing is that sometimes, even though we would rather clean up after a herd of sick elephants than have sex with someone, we still find the pressure from them or the expectations of others intimidating.

Respect!

It is important to understand that you own your body. If people really like you, and do not just want to use you, then they will respect this. They will not do anything without your consent. They won't push you into doing anything you don't want to do, or are not ready for. Because sex is something special, we should be careful not to allow people to abuse it, or us.

It is important to take decisions early on. The problem is that, if you're not going out with someone, or have never gone out with someone – or if you're going out with someone but sex is not yet on the agenda – you might think that it's a bit early to set your standards and make any firm decisions about what you would and wouldn't do when, where and with whom.

But 'waiting until it happens' can prove to be disastrous. If the moment is strong enough, you can end up undressed and losing your virginity – or making the same mistake you made in your last relationship, and promised yourself you would never make again – before you really know what is going on.

Remember that, if you're relying on the telephone ringing, or the CD needing to be changed, or your boyfriend or girlfriend suddenly changing their mind, or your parents returning home unexpectedly, or the Pope appearing to you in a vision and warning you against the error you're just about to make – *anything* to save you having to make a decision yourself – you are likely to be very disappointed.

I used to be indecisive, but now I'm not so sure

You have to make your own decisions about your body. And you need to think about these decisions carefully.

It's the same if you decide to have sex with your boyfriend or girlfriend now, or in the future when your relationship is more established, or to put off having sex until you're married. You need to be clear in your own mind *why* you have made this decision. Because whichever you choose, you will have to live with the consequences. Whatever you decide, you will relive this decision over and over again in the years to come. So make sure that you make the right one.

If you decide to have sex early on in a relationship and it then breaks up – or you meet someone you feel you want to make a long-term commitment to – you may well regret having gone so far now.

And if you decide *not* to have sex outside of a permanent and committed loving relationship, or before marriage, you will almost certainly have to learn to defend this decision not only to a boyfriend or girlfriend, but also to the wider circle of your friends.

It is hard to defend a decision when you don't really know why you made it in the first place.

Some friend YOU are

Friends don't always agree with one another. Although all friendships depend on friends having something in common, no two friends agree on absolutely everything. It can be clothes. Or music. Or opinions. Or sex.

But whilst they may well disagree with one another, sometimes very strongly, true friends nevertheless support and respect each other.

Most of society teaches that sex is a go-ahead-and-do-it kind of thing, without any serious consequences – 'anywhere, any time, any partner, just so long as you use a condom'. This means it's tough to go against the flow and decide *not* to have sex. And if your friends know that you have decided not to have sex as soon or as often as possible, you might find that thay take the mickey out of you a little.

People often find differences of opinion quite threatening, especially if they're not sure of their own opinions. But sometimes, even when your friends take the mickey out of you for what you believe, they secretly admire and respect your stand. They may be influenced by it themselves. They may even agree with you, but lack the courage to say so in public.

So if you've decided not to have sex with your boyfriend or girlfriend at the moment, or not to 'do it' outside of marriage, you can occasionally find yourself the butt of some pretty cruel jokes. The pressure will be on for you to conform.

And unfortunately, although your friends should respect your decisions – even if they think you're wrong, or just plain weird – it doesn't always work out that way. Which is why it's very important to be clear in your own mind about why you've made your decision.

The death of the Lone Ranger

Of course, it helps to have support. It's very hard to go it alone, to stand by a decision you feel is right when everyone else seems to feel that it's wrong. In fact, unless you can leap buildings in a single bound and fly faster than a speeding bullet, it's pretty much impossible. Which is why it is important to find people who have made the same decision.

If your friends can't support you, perhaps it's time to find some additional friends who can, and who understand how difficult it can be for you to stick by your decision, because they're going through the same thing as well.

Alcoholics often find it impossible to give up drinking alone. They need the help and support of others who know what they're going through, and who can understand and anticipate their problems because they've been through the same thing themselves.

Although, for most people, the desire for sex is not as intense as an alcoholic's desire for drink, exactly the same principle applies. It's easier to say 'No' with the support of other people than it is to say 'No' alone.

The best people to give you this kind of support are people who are going through the same difficulties and the same temptations. If you know people like this, people you trust, then make use of them. You can often be as helpful to them as they are to you. If you don't yet know people like this, stay on the lookout. The chances are that they're merely timid about coming out of the woodwork.

At the eleventh hour

It's never too late to make the decision not to have sex.

Some people have sex because they feel that, having got to a certain point, they don't have the right to back out. Perhaps they have been swept along by passion, much further than they would have liked. They want to stop, but feel that it wouldn't now be fair to their partner. Or they just don't know how to call a halt. Or perhaps, having agreed to have sex with someone, they feel that they have to go through with it. It may even have been their idea in the first place.

Always remember that, whatever situation you are in, it is *never* too late to say 'No'. You can change your mind about having sex at *any* time. Even halfway through, if things have got that far. It's your *right* to do so. Never go through with something if you don't really want to.

So what do you do? How do you say 'No'? It's probably best to stop short of the ice-pick-through-the-chest approach. Simply shout (just to make absolutely sure that your partner actually hears), *'Stop! I don't want to do this any more.'* And, if necessary, disentangle yourself.

The chances are that they won't be too pleased. They may even need some convincing that you are serious. But if they respect you, they will stop.

Second-hand goods?

If you've said 'Yes' once, it can be difficult to justify to yourself how or why you should say 'No' another time. After all, if you've already lost your virginity, isn't the damage done?

Well, although your virginity is something that you can only give away once (and should therefore do only after thinking it all through very carefully), it is important to understand that you can always begin again.

If you feel trapped by your past, and think that just because you've had sex you might as well *keep* having it, even though you'd really rather not, then the truth is that your past is controlling you and the choices you are making now. But it shouldn't be that way; you needn't let it be.

Sex matters, because it's a part of who you are; and you matter. You should therefore be in control. Don't think of yourself as soiled or second-hand goods. If people really care about you, they will forgive your past mistakes (even if you still have to live with the consequences). So don't dwell in the past; learn from it, and move on. You can begin again.

'It's good to talk'

Sometimes, however, the element of control is taken away from us. This happens with rape and sexual abuse. We make our decisions clear, but people violate them anyway.

Often people who have been raped or abused feel guilty: they feel that it was their fault, and that there must have been something more they could or should have done to stop what happened to them. But this is *not* the case.

The aim of a rapist or an abuser is to make us feel as though we do not control what we do with our bodies, and that we do not have the right to say 'No'. If you've been abused, or if someone has had sex with you against your will, then you should understand that you're *not* to blame. You're *not* 'dirty'.

It is very important, however, that you tell someone what has happened to you. If you've been abused, the chances are that the person who abused you insisted that you should never tell anyone else. 'It's our little secret.' Perhaps they said that terrible things would happen if you did tell anyone: that no one would believe you, or that they would accuse you of being to blame. If they're a relative, they may even have said that if you told anyone, it would break up the family.

But it's not good to bottle it up inside. It will help a lot to talk about it to someone. This should be someone who has been professionally trained to understand what you've been through and to help you to come to terms with it. But if you don't know anyone like this, it's a good idea to start by telling someone you trust, who can help you to find professional help.

At the back of this book is a list of organisations you can contact for help if you've been abused. You can be sure that they will treat what you have told them in strict confidence, and they will not condemn you for what has happened.

It is not a sign of weakness to seek help. It will be scary, and probably very painful to talk about what has happened to you. But it is the *only* way to be free of it, and to begin again.

The last word

Sex is important. It is not just a physical thing: it's about more than just bonking. It says something basic about who we are as people. Sex is part and parcel of our relationships. It reveals a lot about how much we value ourselves, and how much we value others. It's about showing someone else that we love them, and that we're prepared to be intimate and vulnerable with them.

So the message is this: whether you've been raped or abused, have had sex with your full consent, or have never had sex in your life, it is your *right* to choose when and with whom to have sex in the future. It is a choice which you should make carefully, fully considering all the facts and possible consequences.

Sex is part of who you are. *You* should therefore be in control.

Questions

- Do you think people really feel in control of when and where they have sex?
- Why do you think people feel trapped and guilty if they have been raped or abused?
- Do you think that it's good to wait until you get married to have sex, or not? Why?

14

'Everything you ever wanted to know about sex but were afraid to ask': Sexual terms used in this book

We didn't sit down to write an *A to Z of Sex*. But in case you're not sure what some of the words we've used mean, here's a list of them, with their meanings explained.

Abortion
The termination of a pregnancy. About 15 per cent of all pregnancies end in a 'miscarriage', where a woman's body naturally rejects the foetus growing inside her womb. Sometimes, however, a doctor will end a pregnancy artificially before the foetus is fully grown. This is known as 'abortion'. In the UK it is legal for a woman to have an abortion at any time in the first 24 weeks (six months) of pregnancy if a doctor considers that she might suffer emotionally or physically more by having the baby. Most abortions happen in the first 12 weeks.

Adultery
Sex between two people when at least one of them is married, but not to the person with whom they are having sex.

AIDS
Acquired Immune Deficiency Syndrome. This is the condition, caused by the virus HIV, in which the body's immune system stops working properly. People with AIDS die from diseases which are not lethal for people without AIDS, e.g. pneumonia. Although experts believe that it was around as early as the 1950s, it was not common enough to be properly recognised until 1982. It was first called 'AIDS' in 1983.

Anus
Also called a 'rectum', 'bottom', 'backside' or 'bum'.

Auto-erotic asphyxiation
This is where a person nearly strangles themselves, starving the brain of oxygen, in order to heighten their orgasm. It is extremely dangerous. Too little and you feel nothing; too much and you're dead!

Bisexual
Someone who is sexually attracted to both men and women.

Blow job
The slang term for oral sex.

Bondage
This is where sex involves a relationship of power, one person taking the role of being the 'master' and one being the 'servant'. It often also includes the use of physical restraints such as handcuffs, collars or chains.

Bonking
Slang for sexual intercourse.

Cervix
The cervix is the part of a woman's internal sexual organs where the vagina joins the womb, or 'uterus'.

Chancroid
A bacterial sexually transmitted disease (STD). An ulcer either on the penis or near the vagina, which fills with pus and is very painful. It is cured with antibiotics.

Climax
Another word for orgasm.

Clitoris
This is a small shaft, rather like a miniature penis, above the opening to a woman's vagina. Only the top of this shaft can be seen, as a small bump covered with skin. When a woman is sexually aroused, the clitoris grows and becomes more sensitive and more obvious.

Condom
A form of contraception. A rubber sheath designed to fit over the penis or inside the vagina, which stops sperm from entering the vagina itself.

Contraceptive
Something designed to stop sperm from being able to fertilise an egg.

Diaphragm
A form of contraception. A rubber cap placed over the cervix at the far end of a woman's vagina, designed to stop sperm getting from the vagina into the uterus. Used with a spermicide.

Egg
Not the thing you boil for breakfast! Most animals reproduce by means of the male fertilising the eggs of the female. In women, the eggs are produced by the ovaries and fertilised by sperm.

Ejaculate
Sperm is produced by the testes and travels up the penis during a man's orgasm. The sperm is forced out of the end of the penis by muscles contracting, and this is called ejaculation.

Erection
This is when the penis swells, grows, hardens and turns

upward. It is caused by blood rushing into the penis. This can happen either because a man is sexually aroused, or for reasons that have nothing to do with sex. Men get between two to five erections during sleep, for instance, and research suggests that they do not need to be dreaming of sex for this to happen.

Fallopian tubes
The tubes which connect a woman's ovaries to her uterus. In normal pregnancies, this is where the egg is fertilised.

Fertilisation
A single sperm breaks through the lining of the egg, and . . . hey presto! You're pregnant!

Fetish
In sexual terms, a fetish is a person's obsessive preoccupation either with a part of the anatomy or with an inanimate object. People can get fetishes about anything: toes, breasts, panties or French Maid outfits. The obsessive nature of a fetish can mean that people become unable to enjoy sex without these things.

Foetus
When an egg is fertilised, its cells subdivide and reproduce. Cells then specialise, so that different cells develop into different parts of a baby's body. Between the time that

different organs begin to develop and the time a baby is ready to be born, it is called a foetus.

Genitals
A man's penis and testes, or a woman's labia, clitoris and vaginal opening.

Genital chlamydia
A bacterial sexually transmitted disease (STD). The symptoms are very similar in most cases to those of gonorrhoea. Treatment is with antibiotics.

Genital warts
A viral sexually transmitted disease (STD). Soft, painless warts grow on or near a person's genitals. More a nuisance than a problem, they can nevertheless be a factor in the later development of cancer of the cervix or the penis. They can be removed in the same way as other types of wart, but there is no cure for the virus which causes them.

Gonorrhoea
A bacterial sexually transmitted disease (STD), commonly known as 'clap'. Symptoms begin with a burning sensation when passing urine, and the production of a yellowish liquid which seeps from the opening of the urethra (the tube which takes urine from the bladder to outside the body). If untreated, it can sometimes spread back up the body to cause inflammation of the prostate gland in men or pelvic inflammatory disease in women. Treated with antibiotics.

Grope
To feel or fondle another person's sexual organs.

Heavy petting
Petting is when two people caress each other's bodies. 'Heavy' petting is when this becomes more intense, and attention is focused particularly on each other's genitals. It can be done naked or with clothes on, and often involves 'mutual masturbation'.

Herpes
A viral sexually transmitted disease (STD). Skin around the genitals begins to itch and burn before clear blisters appear, sometimes accompanied by headaches, fever and muscle aches. Symptoms normally disappear within three weeks, but the virus remains dormant inside the body, and can recur at any time. There is no cure.

Heterosexual
Someone who is sexually attracted to people of the opposite sex.

HIV
A viral sexually transmitted disease (STD), the Human Immunodeficiency Virus, which can take years to show itself after a person is infected. HIV invades and destroys the human immune system, which normally helps people to fight off diseases. It is the cause of AIDS.

Homosexual
Someone who is sexually attracted to people of their own sex.

Hormones
Chemicals within the body which are released to stimulate cells into action. Sex hormones are responsible for the changes a person's body undergoes during puberty, but they also keep these changes stable.

Insemination
The process by which sperm is deposited in the uterus and a woman's egg is fertilised.

Intra-uterine device
A T-shaped, plastic and copper contraceptive device, placed inside the uterus to stop a fertilised egg from attaching itself to the walls of the uterus (which it must do if it is to develop into a foetus).

Labia
These are the fleshy 'lips' which surround the opening to a woman's vagina.

Masturbation
This is the stimulation of a person's sexual organs, usually by hand and alone. It is normally done to produce an orgasm, and, in the case of men, results in ejaculation. 'Mutual masturbation' is when two people stimulate each

other's genitals, either instead of or as well as what is called 'penetrative' sexual intercourse (where a man inserts his penis into a woman's vagina).

Menstruation

Otherwise known as a woman's 'period'. One egg is released from one ovary every month. It travels down the Fallopian tube to the uterus. If it is fertilised, it grows into a foetus. If not, it is expelled, together with some blood and the lining of the uterus. This usually lasts a few days, and is sometimes painful.

Morning sickness

During pregnancy, especially in the early stages, some women wake up feeling ill and needing to vomit.

Oral sex

This is where one person stimulates another person's sexual organs with their mouth, often to produce an orgasm in the other person. If a woman licks or sucks a man's penis or testicles, it is called 'fellatio', or more commonly a 'blow job'. If a man licks or sucks a woman's clitoris or labia, it is called 'cunnilingus'.

Orgasm

Also called 'coming' (or 'cumming') or a 'climax'. An orgasm is a set of involuntary muscle spasms caused by stimulating a person's sexual organs. Orgasms can vary in intensity, from mildly pleasant to exhaustingly wonderful. Men usually have an orgasm during sex. Some women rarely or never have an orgasm during sex, whilst others can have two or three in a row.

Ovaries
These are the organs which produce the eggs needed for sexual reproduction. There is one on either side of the uterus. Once a month, hormones instruct one ovary to produce one egg.

Pelvic inflammatory disease
A bacterial sexually transmitted disease (STD), most often caused by either gonorrhoea or chlamydia, in which the Fallopian tubes are infected and can be scarred. It can also cause an abscess (pus-filled swelling) in the ovaries or Fallopian tubes, and pain during sex. Treatment is usually with antibiotics. Pelvic inflammatory disease increases the risk of infertility and an 'ectopic' pregnancy (one in which the foetus grows outside the womb).

Penis
The male sexual organ, used both for sex and for urinating. In males past the age of puberty, it is usually limp, but becomes hard and erect when a man is 'turned on' (sexually aroused). It contains no bone. Some men brag about the size of their penis, whilst others worry. But the truth is that it makes no difference to sexual performance or satisfaction. There are probably more slang words for penis than any other word in the English language!

Pornography
Sexually explicit pictures or text designed to turn someone on without any interest in the person or persons involved.

Promiscuity
Having sex with a number of different people.

Puberty
The stage in a young person's life when they change physically and emotionally from being a boy or girl into being a man or woman. The shape of the body changes and hair starts to grow under the arms, around the genitals, and on the legs. Girls develop breasts and begin to menstruate. Boys start having erections and growing beards, and their voices drop. It can happen quickly or slowly, any time between the ages of about 11 and 18. Girls tend to reach puberty before boys.

Rape
Sexual intercourse when a person is forced to have sex against their will.

Sado-masochism
A sadist is someone who enjoys inflicting pain on others. A masochist is someone who enjoys having pain inflicted on themselves. Sado-masochism, or 'S&M', involves one person causing another pain by arrangement during sex, often by spanking or whipping.

Scrotum
The skin sack containing a man's testicles, situated just below the penis.

Semen
The milky fluid ejaculated by a man during orgasm, containing sperm and nutrients to keep sperm alive for a short while.

Sperm
The cells produced by a man's testes for reproduction. Sperm cells have tails to enable them to swim through the vagina and the uterus, and into the Fallopian tubes in order to fertilise a woman's egg. Although about 100 million sperm are released from the penis into the vagina per ejaculation, only a couple of hundred make it to the Fallopian tubes, and only one fertilises an egg.

Spermicide
A chemical substance designed to kill sperm, used as a contraceptive.

Syphilis
A bacterial sexually transmitted disease (STD). Early symptoms are hard but painless ulcers around the genital region. If untreated, this can develop into the presence of a fever, headache, sore throat and skin rashes. Symptoms then seem to go away, but in one-third of cases come back, sometimes doing serious damage to the heart or the nervous system. Treatment is with penicillin.

Termination
The medical term used for abortion is 'termination' or 'termination of pregnancy'.

Testes
Also called the 'testicles' or 'balls', these are the organs in a man's body which manufacture sperm. The normal temperature of the body is too high for sperm to stay alive, so the testes hang in the scrotum, outside the main structure of the body.

Tubal ligation
This is the process in which the Fallopian tubes connecting the ovaries to the uterus are cut. It is a permanent form of contraception, otherwise known as 'female sterilisation'.

Uterus
The technical term for what we usually call the 'womb'. This is the internal cavity in which a fertilised egg develops into a foetus, and a foetus develops into a baby ready to be born. The uterus stretches and expands during pregnancy.

Vagina
The tube-shaped canal which connects a woman's vulva to her uterus.

Vas deferens
These are the tubes which connect a man's testes to his penis. Sperm produced in the testes must travel along these to get to the penis before it can be ejaculated.

Vasectomy
This is when the *vas deferens* are cut. It is a permanent form of contraception.

Virgin
Someone who has never had sex.

Vulva
The external genital area of a woman's body, including the clitoris, the labia, and the opening to the vagina.

Wanking
The slang word for masturbation.

Wet dreams
Otherwise known as 'nocturnal emissions', these are the result of involuntary erections during sleep, when sperm seeps out of the penis. They are common in boys during puberty, but they can happen for a number of reasons during any time in a man's life. They can be accompanied by an orgasm, even though the person is asleep, which are known as 'nocturnal orgasms'. Women can also get nocturnal orgasms, and can find that vaginal fluid leaks out during sleep or even when they are awake. This is quite normal.

Womb
The common word for uterus.

15

Getting help

General help
This book is unlikely to have answered all your questions about sex and relationships. If you feel that you can't talk to your parent or parents, but you still want to know more about any of the things we've mentioned, you should be able to get help from:

Your school or college. They may have a trained counsellor you can talk to in complete confidence. If they are not qualified to help you with your particular problem, they can refer you to someone who is. That's why they're there.

Your local GP, who can give you confidential medical advice about pregnancy, disease and contraception. They can also point you in the direction of someone to talk to if you are confused or need help.

Help if you have been abused
If you have been abused or taken advantage of, then you

will need to talk to someone who understands what you're going through and is prepared to listen. You can get help and advice from your *school* or your *local GP*. But you can also get confidential help from the following three helplines. Each has people who are trained to listen and to offer advice:

Childline:
A 24-hour national helpline set up to help you if you are the victim of rape, or of any kind of abuse and neglect.
Phone 0800 1111. Calls are free, and they will not show up on the telephone bill.

NSPCC Child Protection Helpline:
Another 24-hour helpline for the victims of abuse, run by the National Society for the Prevention of Cruelty to Children.
Phone 0800 800500. Calls are free, and they will not show up on the telephone bill.

The Samaritans:
provide a listening ear and advice, 24 hours a day, especially when things are desperate (although you don't need to be thinking about committing suicide to call).
Phone 0345 909090. Calls are charged at the local rate.